A GUIDANCE TO MENTAL TRAINING

Learn How to Develop Mental Resilience

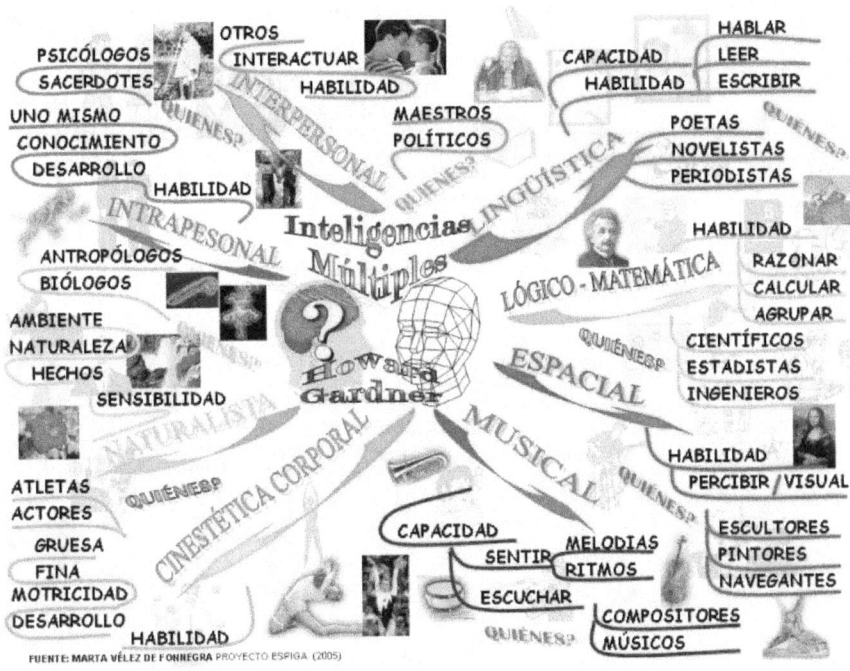

FUENTE: MARTA VÉLEZ DE FONNEGRA PROYECTO ESPIGA (2005)

By Patricia A Carlisle

Introduction

I want to thank you and congratulate you for choosing the book, *"A GUIDANCE TO MENTAL TRAINING: Learn How To Develop Mental Resilience"*.

This book contains proven steps and strategies on how to add Mental Resilience in your life.

Building mental resilience is important if you want to get tougher and build a shield against all the stress and bad things in the world. It is so easy to give up under high pressure and let go of your dreams and hopes for the future.

However, do not despair. There are ways to practice your mental resilience and become a stronger person. Your mind is just like any part of your body. For example, if you want to build muscle, you have to work out a lot of hours. This is almost the same thing. Instead of training the muscles, you are training your brain.

Thanks again for choosing this book, I hope you enjoy it!

TABLE OF CONTENT

Chapter 1

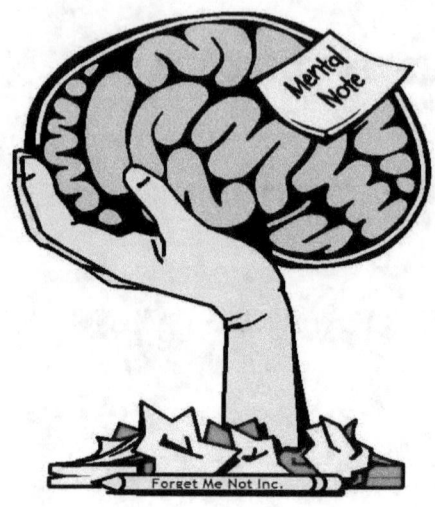

HOW TO STAY FOCUSED ON YOUR GOALS

Mental resilience is the ability to stay on the right path even if life gets difficult. This toughness will also provide you with the strength you need to keep your emotions in check whenever something very bad happens in your life. As an example, if you lose someone you love, you can easily lose yourself too.

An efficient way to help develop your brain is to stay focused on your goals and set up schedules you can stick to no matter what happens. Ask your friends and family to help you out. You can make it like a game. Ask them to come up with all kind of distractions to see if you can be strong enough to say no. They can organize parties in the middle of the week; they can invite you to concerts, or anything else you would love to do. Make sure you have enough things on your schedule to fill your days. Do not let yourself get weak. This is just a game; however, it will help you strengthen your ambition for the future. Life is filled with temptations, and if you are not prepared, you might find it extremely hard to stay focused, and succeed.

Make sure you have realistic expectations for yourself. If your plan is to do a lot in a short period of time, you will end up getting disappointed. Failing to achieve your expectations, can make you feel your are out of control. Things can get overwhelming and distract you from your plans. Make a clear plan for yourself. Write down everything you want to do step by step. Make sure you can manage and change your goals if necessary. Having the power to adapt in different situations is not a weakness. Life is full of surprises, and you should know how you can handle different situations that come your way. Imagine how boring life would be if we could be sure of everything. Sometimes, a little mystery can make things more exciting. Have the power to change things in your favor. Do not allow the lack of control to diminish your morale.

Whatever you do, do not let anything diminish your self-confidence. If something unexpected happens, take a few minutes to think. It is okay to get into panic mode, but only for a few minutes. Do not act impulsively because you might regret it later. You can even pretend that you are giving yourself advice. If there is no one around, you can talk to yourself, and try to think of the pros and cons for each situation. By doing this little exercise, you will detach yourself from the emotional side of the situation. With a cool mind it is much easier to move past anything. If it helps, take a piece of paper, and write your thoughts down. You will see that by doing this, it will be a lot easier to make the right decision. No matter what happens, you have no choice but to pick up the pieces, and move on.

Chapter 2

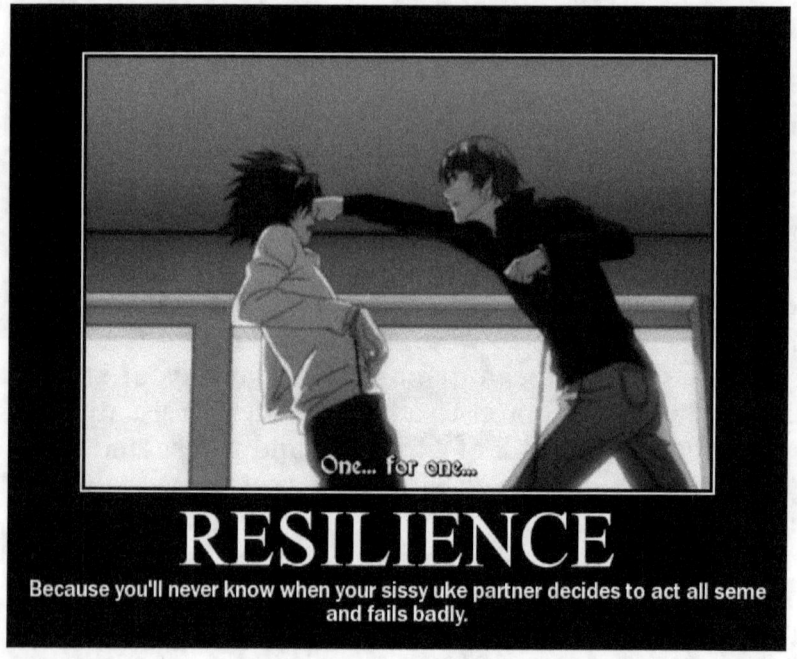

One... for one...

RESILIENCE

Because you'll never know when your sissy uke partner decides to act all seme and fails badly.

HOW TO CONTROL YOUR EMOTIONS

Whenever something emotional happens, you can feel that your judgment is getting clouded. The best way to avoid this is by keeping a cool head. Of course, this is easier said than done. You have to practice getting comfortable with uncomfortable situations. The first step is to accept the reality, and try to deal with it. Your first impulse will be to run away to a safe place. However, you cannot run away from yourself and your emotions. You need to get use to what just happened to you, and try to find the best solution for the future.

Use critical thinking, and start to trust yourself and your instincts. When something really bad happens, the easiest thing you can do is to blame someone else. As you probably know, this is the biggest mistake you can do. Even if someone else is to blame, there is nothing anyone can do. Unfortunately, time cannot be turned back. Being in touch with your emotions is okay as long as you do not let them control your life. A good method to deal with pain is to have your loved ones around you. There is nothing better than having their support no matter what happens to you. Look around you, and try to see who is there for you. Usually, the people you can trust are your friends and family.

Some people keep their feelings bottled up for a long time. By doing this, you are only delay the real solution to the problem. The first thing you should do when something really bad happen is to talk about it with someone you trust. This is how we develop mental resilience. You need to feel the pain and overcome it. Allow yourself a few moments, or even days to get overwhelmed by your emotions. Be sure to put an expiration date to it. When this time ends, take a deep breath, and use your mental resilience.

When the time expires, count to ten, and take a step back. Look at the problem with a clear and cool mind. Imagine what just happened does not affect you personally. Let your mind imagine you are just a stranger helping someone else. What would you advice that person? How would you help him? If you keep your mind cool you will see the light at the end of the tunnel. You might be surprised of how simple the solution really is.

Chapter 3

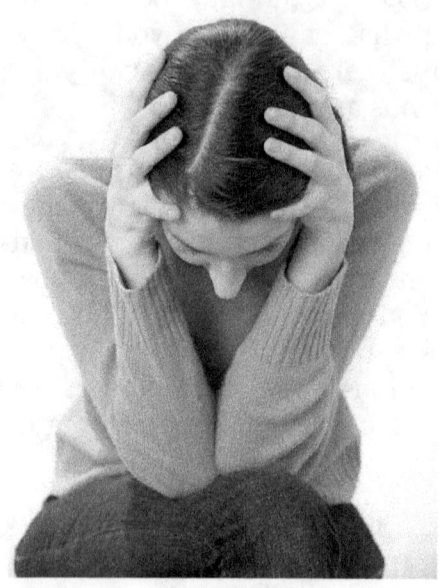

FINDING YOUR MOTIVATION AND STAYING POSITIVE

There is nothing better to build strength and mental resilience than having something that really motivates you. Think about what you want most in this world. As an example, if you have a family, your motivation might be helping your children. You can do this by helping yourself first. Start by finding a better job, and earning more money. There is more to financial wealth then you can imagine. It is not all about money. It is also about the confidence and power it gives you. Trusting yourself is extremely important if you want to become resilient to anything.

A successful career can give you the confidence you need. People will respect you, and this will lead to a boost in your confidence. When you are successful, you are also becoming a good role model for your children. This is something they need in order to build their mental resilience. Before you get to that point, find your own role model in life. This can be anybody. It can be a parent, a teacher, or even some TV star.

If your role model is a person you are in touch with, make sure to talk to him or her as often as possible. It will give you the motivation and strength you need whenever you feel you cannot go on. If your role model is someone you are not in touch with, write down some of his or her achievements, and put them somewhere where you can see them every day. Read the achievement list whenever you feel that you are about to give up.

Face your fears, and tell yourself that you are stronger than anything. Do not hide your head in the sand when something horrible happens to you. Use positive affirmations to try to help you go through them. Whenever you feel down, talk to yourself and try to convince your brain that you can do anything you want. In the end, it is all a matter of believing what you are saying. When you train yourself to trust your abilities, you are halfway there. It will feel like the battle is already won.

Chapter 4

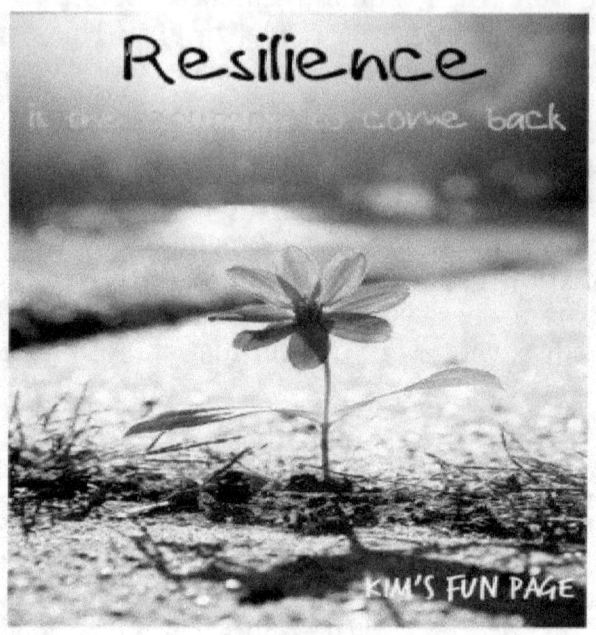

CHALLENGE YOUR MIND

Making sure your mind is always challenged is the next step to creating mental resilience. You can do this by helping others. Try to fix their problems, and imagine those problems are your own. Put yourself into their shoes, and come up with solutions for their problems. By doing this, you are not allowing your brain to take a rest. This is like intensive training for your mind to help keep it strong when you need the mental resilience for your own problems.

If you want to relax, instead of watching TV or playing video games, try reading a good book. This is not just a method to rest your brain. It is a passive way of training your mind for critical thinking. For this purpose, mystery books are the ideal choice.

You can also make up scenarios in your mind. Think about all the things that could happen to you, your family, or your business. Write down all the scenarios in a notebook, and try to find at least two solutions for each possible problem. This will not only prepare you for the worst, but it will also develop a higher strength and ability to cope with negative situations.

Accept that change is a natural part of your destiny. Do not see it as a disaster. If something unexpected and unpleasant occurs, just look at it as a way to prove your strength. In a very bad situation, try to pick the positive things. Maintaining a good attitude is the key to a happy life. It is important to know that being strong does not mean refusing help from the people who love you. Accepting their support is the best thing you can do for yourself and for them. It does not mean you are a weak person it represent strength.

Chapter 5

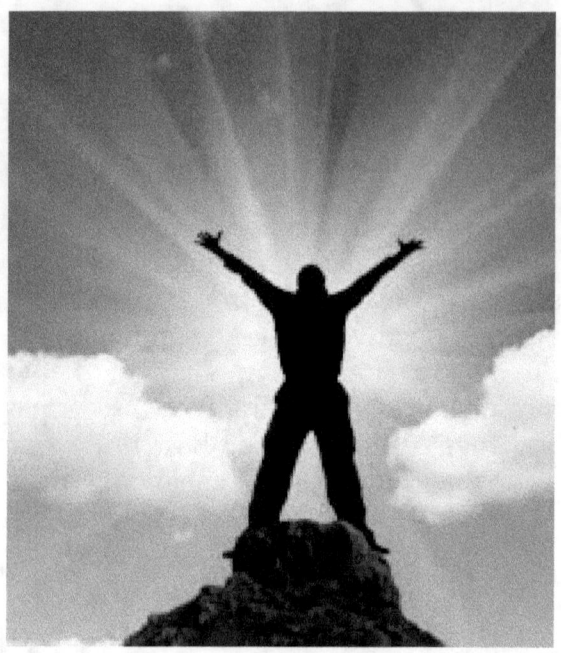

TAKE CARE OF YOURSELF

Your mind is connection to your body. If you are not in perfect physical health, you cannot build mental resilience. This is why you need to make sure you're eating a healthy diet. Exercising your body is also very important. Try to push your limits every time you are exercising. If you love to run, try to lengthen the distance every day. Push past the pain, and try not to give up before the finish line. In sports, you are using your mental resilience more than you can imagine. If you convince yourself that you can go a little longer, you will be pleasantly surprised.

To be prepared for the bad days, you need to enjoy the good days first. This means that you should take advantage of every good thing life has to offer. If you come home after a long day of work, do not start doing house chores. Relax with a cup of hot tea and listen to some good music. Invite your family out for a delicious dinner, or to see a good movie. Make time to have fun with your friends too. Every person is different, and it is up to you to choose the activities that help you relax, and build mental strength. Some people might prefer to be on their own and watch a TV show. Whatever you choose to do, the important thing is to reduce stress.

Do not waste a lot of nights. Having a good rest at night is essential for mental health and resilience. If you have a job where you have to work during the night, try to make up for the lost sleep during the day. Being in a great mental and physical shape is essential for overcoming any hardship you might have in the future.

Building resilience does not mean always thinking of the bad things that might happen. If you do this, you end up wasting the time you could use to enjoy the amazing things that are happening right now in your life. No matter how much you think of the negative things that can happen, you can never be prepared for real life surprises. If you spend your time enjoying yourself, your mind will be prepared to face anything that comes your way. Of course you will be shocked some days, and feel your world is crumbling at your feet. This is a perfectly normal reaction. What matters is how you manage the problem and your emotional reactions. This is where the real strength is. The way you respond to high levels of stress shows how strong you really are. Allow yourself to experience all the emotions, but at the same time, do not let your bad feelings affect the decisions you make.

Chapter 6

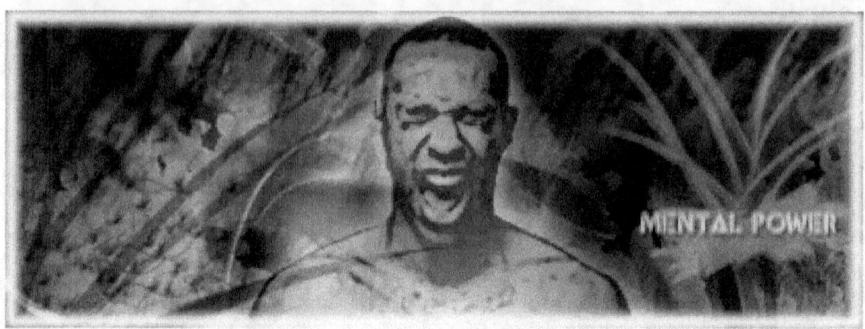

HOW TO DEVELOP CRITICAL THINKING SKILLS

Critical thinking skills are required for achieving your goals in your career, and also in your personal life. There are some excellent ways to develop critical thinking skills. First of all, you need to learn how to use your time wisely. Everybody wastes time every single day without realizing it. There are some people who will jump from one activity to another, and fail to finish a task. You can avoid doing that by trying to be more productive, and using time in your favor. Imagine how many things you could do in a day if you just stay focused. If you finish your work earlier, you can use the time to enjoy yourself and relax. A second strategy for developing critical thinking is solving one problem at a time. Do not allow yourself to get overwhelmed with several problems. When you do this, you end up not having enough time to resolve any of them. Start with the problem that needs to be fixed urgently. You can also leave some problems for the next day. A good night sleep can help you see things clearly.

People can change if that is what they really want. You can reshape your character the way you want. Each week, you should work on a certain character trait. Start with the traits you feel needs the most improvement. For example you can work on your perseverance and courage. Next, redefine the way you see a problem. The way you look at something reflects not just the way you feel about it but also how you solve the problem.

You can change the way you see things by training your mind to see things in a positive light. Ask yourself "how can I turn a negative situation into a positive one?" At a first glance, you might think it is impossible to see anything positive from a certain problem. However, this is not true. For example, if a good friend betrayed your trust, you can learn from that experience and in the future you will be able to choose your friends carefully. If you open your mind, you can always learn something useful that can lead to a better future.

Chapter 7

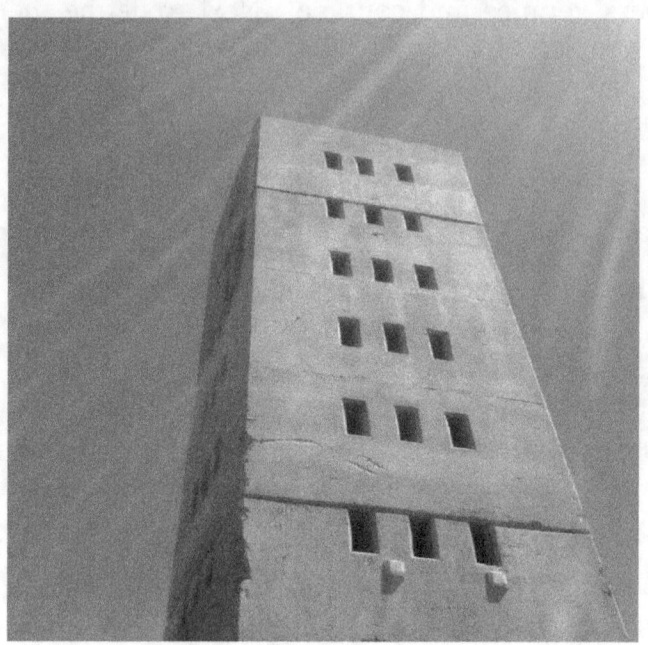

CONSERVE YOUR MENTAL ENERGY

You can easily spend all your mental energy by focusing on things you cannot change. Instead of thinking of negative things, try to focus on what can be done. For example, if your hear a major storm is coming, instead of trying to find a way to stop it, focus on what you can do to protect yourself and your home. Your mental energy should be used only for productive tasks. This involves setting goals and making an effort to use your mental energy for productive things.

Imagine a box where you can put all the things that cannot be changed. Put everything that cannot be changed and forget about that box ,and try to use your mind for the things that can be changed. Whenever you have some free time, learn how to meditate. This is a very efficient way to relax your mind, and work on your ability to focus. Meditation is a way to clear your mind and relief all the stress from your life. In today's world it is very difficult to relax and forget about the day-to-day stress. This is way practicing meditation is very important. It will give your mind a break from everything, and will help to recharge its energy.

Your mental energy should be used to practice tolerance to discomfort. Having mental resilience does not mean avoiding emotions. It is actually the opposite. It means accepting that a situation brings you a strong discomfort and negative feelings. What is important is how you deal with it. You need to push through the discomfort. To do this, you will need courage and resilience.

Note your progress every day. It is easy to look back and have the feeling you made no progress. It is important to record every little success you have. Imagine you suffer from social anxiety. If one day you manage to stay for an hour in a crowded mall, you can consider that a victory. You will have days when your feel like giving up. During those bad days, it is important to look back on your achievements. It will give you enough motivation to move past the depression.

Conclusion

Thank you again for choosing this book!

I hope this book was able to help you to mentally train you mind.

Mental resilience is not something just for military people. You can use it in your day to day life. It is the mental strength that pushes you forwards no matter how many challenges you face in life.

Keep a positive attitude and follow your dreams no matter what. The real strength of a person in not measured in the size of his or her success, but in the way they manages to get up whenever life knocks them down.

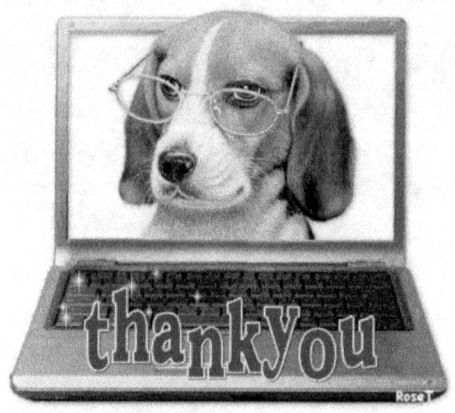

Finally, if you enjoyed this book, be kind enough to leave a review for this book on Amazon? It'd be greatly appreciated!

Thank you and good luck!

Preview Of 'MINDFULNESS EXERCISES FOR BEGINNERS'

Chapter 1
WHAT IS MINDFULNESS

So what does it mean to be mindful? As a child I was occasionally told, -Mind your manners! This mean I should be aware of what I was doing and how it was affecting other people-usually adults! That's not a bad start; mindfulness certainly is about paying attention. Paying attention to what is happening right now, right before our eyes-and ears and nose and other senses, including our internal ones. Also, what pains and tensions are there in our body, how are you feeling right now, are you aware of what you are thinking or are you on automatic, daydreaming, or perhaps going over and over a difficult encounter? Many of the problems mentioned above relate to the future or the past. Anxiety and stress can result from worrying about future events. Depression is often associated with replaying past events in our mind. We go over past are events or we are anxious about the future.

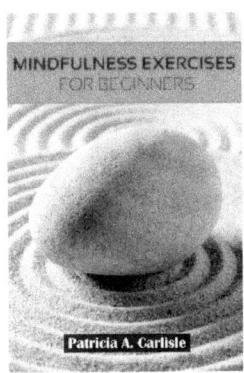

Mindfulness Exercises For Beginners.

Check Out My Other Books

Below you'll find some of my other popular books that are popular on Amazon and Kindle as well. Alternatively, you can visit my author page on Amazon to see other work done by me. (https://amazon.com/author/patriciacarlisle)

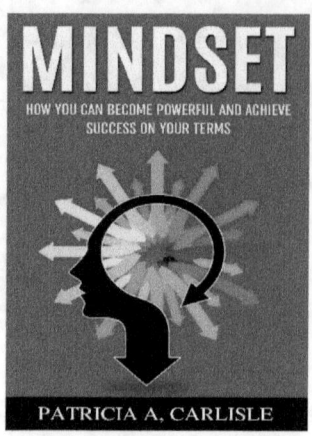

MINDSET: HOW YOU CAN BECOME POWERFUL AND ACHIEVE SUCCESS ON YOUR TERMS.

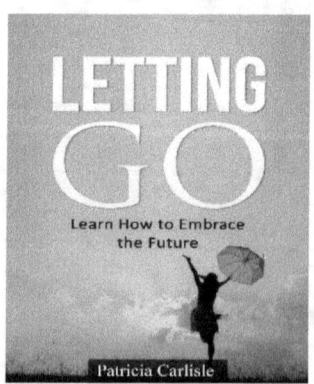

LETTING GO: LEARN HOW TO EMBRACE THE FUTURE.

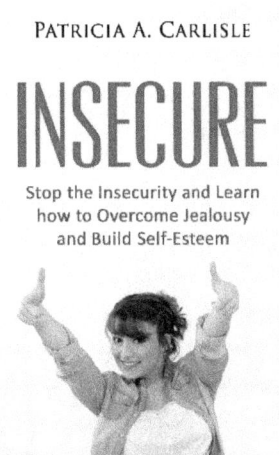

Insecure: Stop the Insecurity and Learn How to Overcome Jealousy and build Self Esteem.

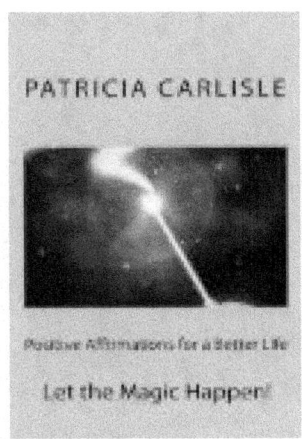

POSITIVE AFFIRMATIONS FOR A BETTER LIFE: LET THE MAGIC BEGIN!

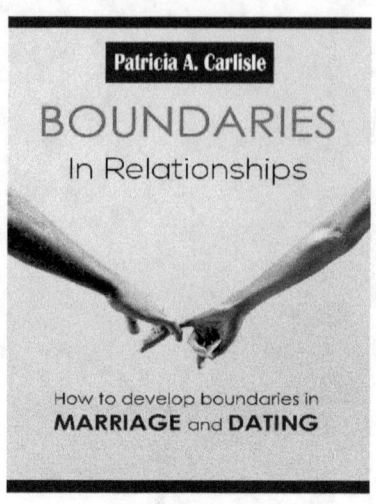

**BOUNDARIES IN RELATIONSHIPS: HOW TO DEVELOP
BOUNDARIES IN MARRIAGE AND DATING.**

You can simply search for these titles on the Amazon website
to find them.

BONUS: SUBSCRIBE TO THE FREE
BOOK

Beginners Guide to Yoga & Meditation

> "Stressed out? Do You Feel Like The World
> Is Crashing Down Around You? Want To
> Take A Vacation That Will Relax Your Mind,
> Body And Spirit? Well this Easy To Read
> Step By Step E-Book Makes It All Possible!"

So many people have achieved a sense of wellness they have never felt before just through a few short yoga sessions. **You can Download my FREE BOOK inside any of my Kindle ebooks**

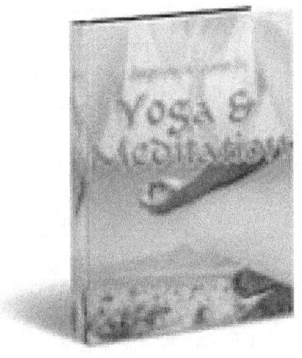
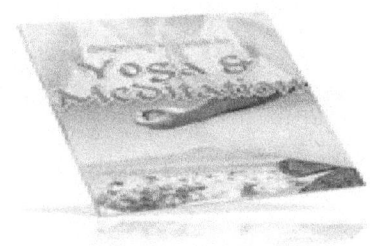

NOTES

NOTES

NOTES

NOTES

NOTES

NOTES

NOTES

NOTES

NOTES

NOTES

www.ingramcontent.com/pod-product-compliance
Lightning Source LLC
Chambersburg PA
CBHW061938280526
45787CB00004B/1649